# SYMPTOMS AND CAUSES OF EMOTIONAL AND PHYSICAL STRESS.

## Unveiling the basic causes of stress.

By

## Dr DOUGLAS JASON

Before this document is duplicated or reproduced in any manner, the publisher's consent must be gained.

Therefore, the contents within can neither be stored electronically, transferred, nor kept in a database. Neither in part nor in full can the document be copied, scanned, faxed, or retained without approval from the publisher or creator.

**TABLE OF CONTENT**

**ABOUT THE AUTHOR**

**INTRODUCTION**

**TABLE OF CONTENTS**

# CONCLUSIONS

## ABOUT THE AUTHOR

Dr. Douglas Jason is a certified dietician who has a strong passion for wellness and a big eagerness to help people all over the world. He uses healthy food, herbs, spices, and other useful tools to help mankind realize its overall goal of optimum health.

## INTRODUCTION

What Stress Indicators Are Physical and Emotional? Definition Causes Symptoms When to Visit a Physician Diagnoses and Therapies

What exactly is stress?
Stress is a state of emotional or physical tension that results from facing a task, demand, or threat. These stimuli cause physical and emotional responses in your body.

Our behavior and attitude can be affected in several ways by stress. The body's numerous systems, organs, and tissues are all affected by stress.

# CHAPTER 1

## SIGNS OF STRESS, BOTH PHYSICAL AND EMOTIONAL

The cardiovascular system, digestive system, immune system, endocrine system, muscular system, reproductive system, and respiratory system are among the bodily symptoms of stress. Anxiety, despair, feeling overburdened or unmotivated, irritability or moodiness, loneliness, and isolation are some of the emotional symptoms of stress.

# CHAPTER 2

## SIGNS AND SYMPTOMS OF STRESS

Stress symptoms and signs Your entire body is impacted by stress, which manifests as several physical ailments. These body systems exhibit tangible signs of stress:

circulatory system
Stress frequently triggers your body's "fight or flight" reaction, during which stress hormones like cortisol, noradrenaline,

and adrenaline raise your heart rate. The heart muscle contracts more forcefully while under stress. Additionally, the blood arteries that supply the heart and big muscles with blood enlarge, raising your blood pressure and raising your risk of suffering a heart attack or stroke.

intestinal system
Your liver will create more blood sugar (glucose) when you're under stress to provide you with more energy. Your

chance of getting type 2 diabetes may rise as a result of this blood sugar surge over time.

An increase in heart rate, fast breathing, and stress hormones can all disturb your digestive tract. Constipation, diarrhea, acid reflux, heartburn, cramps, and even nausea and vomiting are possible symptoms.

system of defense

Your immune system may become weakened over time by stress chemicals. Chronic stress makes you more prone to viral infections and other ailments.

hormone system
The hypothalamic-pituitary-adrenal (HPA) axis is involved in a series of processes that are triggered when your brain detects a threat. As a result, there is an increase in the synthesis of steroid hormones,

such as cortisol, the main stress hormone.

skeletal system
Your muscles may stiffen up when you're under stress. Although muscles tend to loosen up when stress levels decrease, people who are continuously stressed may always be tense.

Reproductive technique
Male testosterone production may increase under short-term

stress. Chronic stress, on the other hand, might result in a drop in testosterone, which may lead to erectile dysfunction or lower sperm production. The risk of infection in the male reproductive system may also rise as a result of ongoing stress.

# CHAPTER 3

## WOMENS' MENSTRUAL CYCLES AND STRESS.

Stress can have an impact on a woman's menstrual cycle by making her periods heavier, more irregular, or uncomfortable. Additionally, persistent stress may make menopause symptoms worse. Stress can have an impact on conception issues as well as the pregnancy process.

respiratory apparatus
You'll probably breathe more quickly when under stress. Your body is seeking to swiftly circulate oxygen-rich blood throughout your body, which is why this happens. You can find it difficult to manage the additional lung strain if you already have a respiratory disorder, such as asthma.

# CHAPTER 4

## EMOTIONAL SIGNS AND STRESS ARE CAUSED

Numerous emotional symptoms can be brought on by chronic stress, which can also harm your physical and mental health. The following are some emotional signs of ongoing stress:


Easily irritated or depressed
Anxiety\sDepression

feeling overburdened or
uninspired
Isolation and solitude


stress factors
Stressors are considered to be
outside influences and are
situations or occurrences that
lead to stress. Internal issues,
such as how you interpret and
interpret your circumstances,
can also contribute to stress.

the following are typical outside factors that generate stress:

your work or studies
your ties to family and friends
money situation
Your place of residence
Your timetable

The following are typical internal stressors:

rigidity or a lack of suppleness in thought
Low self-esteem or negative self-talk
Pessimism or negativity
Perfectionism
a need for certainty or incapacity to deal with unpredictability
It's vital to remember that everyone experiences pressures differently. One person's unpleasant circumstance could be another person's fun or exciting experience.

When should I get a stress checkup?

Your physical or mental health may suffer greatly as a result of stress over time. Contact your doctor if you have attempted to handle your stress on your own but are still having trouble. They might be able to suggest further methods or make a referral to a mental health counselor for additional assistance.

If your stress is making you more likely to use drugs or alcohol or to have suicidal thoughts, call your doctor right away. They can give you advice and resources to manage your stress.

# CHAPTER 5

# STRESS DIAGNOSIS

Identifying stress
Stress is regarded as a disturbance of healthy homeostasis. When under stress, the hypothalamic-pituitary-adrenal (HPA) axis and the sympathoadrenal system both become more active in your body (SAS). This implies that a diagnosis is difficult and dependent on a wide range of variables. Questionnaires, biochemical

measurements, and physiologic procedures are some examples of diagnostic instruments.

# CHAPTER 6

# STRESS REHABILITATION

stress management methods
There are numerous ways to
alleviate stress, including:

Make behavioral adjustments
Put a healthy diet and exercise
first. Eat more fruits and
vegetables, reduce your sugar
intake, and begin an exercise
program that works for your
schedule and level of fitness.

Get rid of the anxiety-causing factors.

If your employment is the source of your stress, you might want to discuss your workload with your boss. When you're already overbooked, start saying "no" to plans if your busyness is causing you to worry. If tough or domineering people in your life are the source of your stress, try talking to them about how they make you feel or avoid them entirely.

Additionally, there are integrative stress management therapies available:

Mindfulness and meditation Meditation is an age-old technique that promotes relaxation by emphasizing breathing and present-moment awareness of the body. A technique called meditation and mindfulness-based stress reduction (MBSR) uses the fundamentals of meditation to make you more conscious of the effects that unfavorable thoughts have on your body. Improved memory and focus, more resilience, and fewer mood fluctuations are some other advantages of MBSR.

Behavioral and cognitive therapy

Talk therapy to recognize and challenge unfavorable or intrusive ideas is known as cognitive behavioral therapy (CBT). According to studies, CBT can be just as helpful as other types of therapy or prescription anti-depressant and anti-anxiety drugs. Additionally, it can support these other therapies.

Acupuncture
A long-standing Chinese custom is an acupuncture. Your immunological and neural systems are stimulated during a session by a certified professional acupuncturist using very few needles. There is proof that acupuncture reduces the body's stress reaction.

Massage

Numerous stress-related conditions, including anxiety and insomnia, can be helped by massage. Stress can be reduced by massage because it boosts endorphins, serotonin, and dopamine. Additionally, massage helps alleviate tight muscles, lower cortisol levels, and improve tissue suppleness.

.

## CONCLUSIONS

When should I get a stress checkup?
Your physical or mental health may suffer greatly as a result of stress over time. Contact your doctor if you have attempted to handle your stress on your own but are still having trouble. They might be able to suggest further methods or make a referral to a mental health counselor for additional assistance.

If your stress is making you more likely to use drugs or alcohol or to have suicidal thoughts, call your doctor right away. They can give you advice and resources to manage your stress.

www.ingramcontent.com/pod-product-compliance
Lightning Source LLC
Chambersburg PA
CBHW071124220526
45467CB00004B/2056